RESISTANT STARCH BIBLE

RESISTANT STARCH - FIBER, GUT HEALTH, GUT BALANCE

Second Edition

CHASE WILLIAMS

© 2015

DISCLAIMER

This book is not intended as a substitute for the medical advice of physicians. The reader should regularly consult a physician in matters relating to his/her health and particularly with respect to any symptoms that may require diagnosis or medical attention.

CONTENTS

INTRODUCTION 5

WHAT, EXACTLY, ARE CARBOHYDRATES?.......................9

WHAT IS FIBER & WHERE DOES IT COME FROM? 13

ISN'T STARCH & FIBER THE SAME THING?.......................15

SO WHAT ARE RESISTANT STARCHES? 17

HOW TO ADD MORE RESISTANT STARCHES TO YOUR DIET 20

CAN RESISTANT STARCH HELP YOU LOSE WEIGHT?.....25

RESISTANT STARCH'S ROLE IN IBS & SIBO 28

RESISTANT STARCH FOR CONSTIPATION 31

RESISTANT STARCH & LEAKY GUT SYNDROME 37

RESISTANT STARCH FOR DIABETES..................................43

CONCLUSION 48

INTRODUCTION

Resistant starch is a popular topic these days, with hundreds of people experimenting with it and seeing major improvements by adding it to their diet. Yet, there is still very little known about resistant starches, such as what they are exactly, what foods they are found in and how specifically they can be of benefit as part of your daily diet.

This book has been written to give you a greater understanding of what resistant starches are, how you can make resistant starches a part of your daily diet and what the actual benefits are of resistant starches on your health and well-being.

In order to achieve this goal I have attempted to use easy to understand terminology, staying away from the scientific jargon so often found in books of this type and scope. Where such jargon is necessary, you will find that I have provided an easy to understand definition, so that you will be able to understand exactly what we are talking about and will not need to be reaching for your dictionary or thesaurus, or looking up terminology online.

While carbohydrates may be a complex subject (no pun intended) you will find that this book presents the subject in such an easy to understand and straight-forward manner that much of the mystery will be taken out of this subject while still providing in depth details on the way your body metabolizes (aka processes) these necessary components of your diet and how you can help your body along by eating the "good" starches while avoiding the "bad" starches.

Before we even begin with this book, let me point out that "resistant starches" are not synonymous with "safe starches". If you've heard the term "safe starches", you might confuse the "good" starches (mentioned above) with this term. However, "safe starches" are an inventive term coined by Drs. Paul and Shou-Ching Jaminet and set forth in "The Perfect Health Diet" (aka PHD).

The Jaminets define "safe starch" as "starchy food which, after normal cooking, lacks toxins, chiefly protein toxins". They encourage people to consume approximately 400 calories per day (or 20% of daily caloric intake) of safe starches and prioritize glucose over fructose. The Jaminets insist that a diet too low in glucose can lead to a variety of health problems such as nutrient deficiencies and kidney stones.

The pros and cons of this concept of "safe starch" is still under debate, but I only include it here to differentiate it from "resistant starch", which has very little to do with the "safe starch" concept. Many opponents of "safe starch" concept have argued that carbohydrates should be avoided as much as possible, but almost all agree that glucose is a necessary component in our daily diet.

The fact is that people do, indeed, need glucose as it supplies energy to the brain as well as making up molecules called "glycoproteins" (simply defined as a protein that contains carbohydrate), which in turn supports a healthy immune system. Of course, diabetics should be especially careful of how they take in their carbs, paying close attention to how certain foods may increase insulin levels, and how some foods (resistant starches in particular) can actually help to level of blood glucose levels. I've included a chapter in this book that deals exclusively with how you can help your diabetes through a good resistant starch diet.

You'll discover in this book how resistant starches cannot only heal your leaky gut and contribute to your overall gut health, but how resistant starch can also help you lose weight, by helping you feel fuller longer and helping you to cut out those frequent in-between snackings that come from eating foods with less satiety. You will learn which foods are the richest in Resistant Starches and how best to prepare your "starchy" foods to bring out the most resistant starches within.

By the time you are finished reading this book, you should be able to consider yourself an expert in the area of resistant starches, to the point where you can explain exactly what resistant starches are and where they come from as well having a complete understanding of the ways in which your body utilizes carbohydrates and the different ways it breaks down starches and resistant starches.

Not only will you understand carbohydrates, starches, fiber and resistant starches but you can help others to understand the benefit of increasing their intake of resistant starches, especially those suffering from gut ailments such as Leaky Gut Syndrome, or those suffering from autoimmune disorders that may arise from imbalance of gut flora. If you, or someone you love is struggling the Type II diabetes, you now have the tools to combat this disease and to level off those pesky blood glucose levels, while increasing your health and decreasing your weight gain. All in all, by the time you have finished reading this book, you will understand precisely why resistant starch is now being touted as a true superfood.

WHAT, EXACTLY, ARE CARBOHYDRATES?

You've no doubt heard of carbohydrates, especially when dealing with diets and weight loss, but few people actually really understand what a carbohydrate is and how it works in our bodies. If you look up the term in an online dictionary or on a wiki, you will probably find the explanation more than a little confounding as it breaks down chemical properties in scientific terms that, to be honest, goes over most people's heads.

In this chapter we will explain in easy to understand terminology exactly what a carbohydrate is and how the body processes different forms of carbohydrates to give us energy and maintain our metabolic processes. A good understanding of carbohydrates is necessary in order to understand how starches are utilized by the body and why resistant starch is of benefit to your daily diet.

Carbohydrates are part of four major classes of biomolecules (which is a fancy term for molecules important to a biological organism, e.g. the human body). The four major classes of biomolecules include proteins, nucleotides, lipids and carbohydrates. Carbohydrates are the most abundant of these four.

The word "Carbohydrate" is derived from the actual composition of carbohydrates; Carbon, Oxygen and Hydrogen.

Carbohydrates come from nearly all foods, with the exception of animal meats and some seafood. Carbohydrates break down into glucose, which is the simplest form of carbohydrates. Glucose is used by your body to provide energy to every living cell in your body. Most of your calories need to come from carbohydrates due to the body's requirement of glucose to produce energy.

There are two types of carbohydrates, simple and complex. Simple carbohydrates include sucrose, lactose and fructose. Complex carbohydrates are organic compounds found in many different foods. All carbohydrates are made up of sugar molecules and whenever three or more of these molecules are bound together it is considered a complex carbohydrate.

Both simple and complex carbohydrates are converted into glucose by your body, but how you digest these carbs is slightly different for each one.

Your body usually uses the glucose it needs from the carbohydrates almost immediately, storing the rest of the glucose in your liver and muscles as glycogen. Glycogen is a complex carbohydrate that your system converts to glucose when carbohydrates from food are unavailable. When your body needs energy to fuel cells, such as when you are doing a rigorous workout, the body will burn stored glycogen, turning it into energy, if you do not have enough carbohydrates readily available. This is why you might feel fatigued early in your workout, especially if you haven't eaten anything recently before the workout. Eating a meal rich in carbohydrates shortly after a workout will help to replace glycogen in your system, so that your body will continue to function at peak performance.

Another word for carbohydrates is saccharides. The various types of saccharides consists of monosaccharides (simple carbohydrates) disaccharides and polysaccharides (complex carbohydrates). The word "saccharide" is from the root "sucre" from which we derive the word "sugar".

Monosaccharides are the smallest possible sugar. Glucose is a monosaccharide, as is fructose and galactose. When we measure blood sugar we are measuring the level of glucose in the blood. As mentioned previously, glucose is the major source of energy for our cells. Fructose is usually found in vegetables and fruits and galactose is found most readily in milk and dairy products.

Disaccharides are made up of two monosaccharides that are bonded together. The suffix "di" means two. Disaccharides can also be considered Polysaccharides as the suffix "poly" means literally two or more. If you bond the monosaccharides fructose and glucose together you will get the disaccharide sucrose, which is commonly found in regular sugar (the kind we use in our coffee). If you bond glucose with galactose you end up with lactose, which is commonly found in milk.

Polysaccharides are made up of a chain of two or more monosaccharides (remember poly means two or more). A Polysaccharide chain may be made up of hundreds or even thousands of monosaccharides. Starch and dietary fiber are the two types of polysaccharides.

There are many foods that contain starch and dietary fiber including bread, cereals and vegetables. Starch is found in potatoes, dry beans, peas and corns as well as cereals and grains. Dietary fiber is in vegetables, fruits, and whole grain foods.

WHAT IS FIBER & WHERE DOES IT COME FROM?

Fiber helps to slow down digestion, which allows foods to break down much slower and not become sugar as quickly. This in turn helps the body to maintain healthy blood sugar levels. The two types of fiber is soluble and insoluble fiber. Soluble simply means easily dissolved. Both soluble and insoluble fiber are undigested, and contain 0 calories. While starch is converted to glucose for energy, fiber does not get converted to energy as it is not absorbed into the bloodstream. Soluble fiber forms a gel while insoluble fiber passes through our intestines pretty much intact.

Fiber encourages the growth of healthful bacteria in our gut. Dietary fiber also helps to regulate your digestive system, and affects the rate at which you absorb certain nutrients.

Soluble fiber helps to slow the digestive process which allows your body to gain the full benefit from the nutrients in the food. Soluble fiber also helps to control the cholesterol in your small intestine, actually lowering the total level of cholesterol in your blood. In particular by minimizing low-density lipoprotein (LDL). Soluble fiber also slows down the absorption of sugar which helps to prevent your blood glucose level from spiking, particularly after a carbohydrate-rich meal.

Fruits and vegetables are rich in soluble fiber, especially citrus fruits such as oranges, lemons and grapefruits. Most berries also contain a high level of soluble fiber, as well. Apples and pears also provide soluble fiber, as do bananas. Peas, lentils and beans are very rich in soluble fiber as are potatoes (both white and sweet). Some grains are also good sources of soluble fiber, such as oats and barley.

Insoluble fiber, also known as roughage, stimulates the activity of your intestines, and helps in digesting your food. Insoluble fiber adds bulk to your stools which helps keep you regular and aids in preventing constipation and other bowel problems. Insoluble fiber can also help in avoiding diverticular disease which is an inflammatory disorder of the intestines.

Most leafy green vegetable such as spinach, collard greens and turnip greens are great sources of insoluble fiber. Other vegetables such as carrots, cabbage, cauliflower and Brussel sprouts also contain insoluble fiber. The peels of most fruits and vegetables also contains a large portion of insoluble fiber, so eating that potato with its skin still on will provide you with both insoluble and soluble fiber alike. You can also get a good dose of insoluble fiber from the peels of apples, pears, peaches, plums and other like fruit. Whole grains (grains with their bran still intact) are an excellent source of insoluble fiber as well, as are breads and cereals made from whole grain flour. Almonds, walnuts and Brazil nuts can also provide you with a good dose of insoluble fibers.

ISN'T STARCH & FIBER THE SAME THING?

Starch is often is confused with fiber. They are both complex carbohydrates and they are both very important for your overall health. The difference between the two, however, is that while fiber is indigestible, starch is usually highly digestible.

Starches are usually found in most root vegetables as well as grains and legumes. As soon as you ingest these starches your body will start digesting them, extracting the nutrients and utilizing the glucose for energy. Starchy foods also contain many nutrients, vitamins, fiber, calcium and iron.

Wholegrain varieties of starchy foods are usually a great source of both starch and fiber. Starch is the most common form of carbohydrate in our diet and we should consume some starchy foods every day as part of a healthy, balanced diet.

Many people believe that starchy foods are too fattening and should be avoided, but the truth of the matter is that starchy foods usually contain less than 50% of their calories from fat. The problem is that many starchy foods are cooked with added fat (such as comes from butter and some types of oils) which increases the overall fat content.

Chemically, starch is a white, odorless and tasteless complex carbohydrate made up of long chains of glucose molecules, especially amylose and amylopectin.

Amylose is a polysaccharide made up of "D-glucose" units (which is a fancy term for dextrose) and composes around 20 to 30 percent of the total structure of starch. Amylopectin composes the remaining 70 to 80 percent and is also a polysaccharide.

The main difference between Amylose and Amylopectin is that Amylose is an un-branched component of starch whereas amylopectin is a branched component. Branched means there are side chain substituents (atoms or groups of atoms replacing other atoms in the molecule) on the longest carbon chain of the molecule. Unbranched means there are no side chain substituents. Therefore, Amylose is insoluble where amylopectin is highly soluble.

The preceding paragraph may be a bit difficult to understand unless you are familiar with chemistry, but what it basically breaks down to is that the Amylose part of starches is not easily digested and behaves quite a bit like fiber in our digestive tracts, whereas the amylopectin breaks down into the smaller molecules of glucose which is more easily absorbed into our blood and immediately available for energy (i.e. turned into glucose).

SO WHAT ARE RESISTANT STARCHES?

A good background understanding of carbohydrates, fiber and starches is necessary to understanding exactly what resistant starches are and how they work. Resistant starches are sometimes referred to the "third type of fiber", where the first two types of fiber are soluble and insoluble fiber. Resistant starch, much like fiber, goes through your digestive tract without being digested and much of it is fermented in the large intestine.

The term "resistant" refers to the starch's ability to resist digestion. Instead of being digested immediately, as regular starch is, it passes through to the large intestine where it acts the same as soluble and insoluble fibers.

Since resistant starch is not fully digested, we extract about 2 calories of energy per gram vs about 4 calories per gram from other starches. This basically means that 100 grams of resistant starch is worth only 200 calories, while the same amount of non-resistant starch will give you 400 calories. So, resistant starch will give you that full filling without actually causing you to put on unwanted weight.

Like other fibers, when resistant starches arrive in the large intestine they act as prebiotic fibers which helps to feed the microbes (microorganisms) that live in your large intestine. Intestinal bacteria ferments resistant starches, producing short-chain fatty acids (SCFAs) and improving the setting for healthful bacteria to flourish.

These healthful bacteria help to produce vitamins as well as aiding in detoxifying (removing harmful toxins) and converting gut bacteria into isothiocyanates. Isothiocyanates are bioactive compounds that actually fight cancer and keep it from being produced or growing in your gut.

There are actually hundreds of different types of bacteria found in the intestine and the number of bacteria as well as the type of bacteria can have a very profound impact on your overall health.

Resistant starch feeds the friendly bacteria in the intestine, having a positive effect on the type of bacteria as well as the number of them.

One of the main reasons why resistant starch improves health, is that it feeds that friendly bacteria in the intestine and increases production of short-chain fatty acids like butyrate.

Butyrate is a remarkable molecule that has been shown to help in stopping cancer and some neurodegenerative diseases (diseases that cause a loss of function in nerves aka nerve degeneration such as Alzheimer's disease or Parkinson's). Butyrate has also been shown to help cure IBS (Irritable Bowel Syndrome).

There are actually 4 different types of resistant starches:

Resistant starch type 1:

This is found in seeds, grains and beans. This type of resistant starch is bound by plant cell walls, which means it resists digestion due to the fact that cell walls are not digestible.

Resistant starch type 2:

This type of resistant starch is found in raw potatoes, unripe bananas and plantains and isn't digestible in its raw state.

Resistant starch type 3 (RS3):

Some starches become harder to digest when heated and then cooled down. This is known as "starch retrogradation", which is basically the structure of the starches changing to become more resistant to digestion. When certain foods are cooked, then cooled, the starch chains slowly bond to each other more tightly.

Resistant starch type 4 (RS4):

This type of resistant starch isn't found in nature, but is a man-made starch, chemically modified to become more resistant.

The two types of starch we will be paying attention to most is Types 2 & 3. You should avoid RS4 completely, as it is really not known what long term effect modified food starch actually has on the body. Type 1 is great, but the actual amount of nutritional resistant starch in most seeds, grains and beans is so small, in order to get enough you would have to eat an excessive amount of the food.

HOW TO ADD MORE RESISTANT STARCHES TO YOUR DIET

The problem with trying to increase your intake of resistant starches is that, unlike many other dietary intake information, resistant starches (or starch in general) are not yet listed on food labels, though sometimes resistant starches are listed as "dietary fiber". There is a way to figure out how much starch a product contains, however, but it requires a little math work on your part.

First, find the total number of grams of carbohydrates on the nutrition facts label. Next, subtract the fiber from the total carbs. This will give you the net carbs per serving. Then, subtract the sugars from the net carbs. Net carbs comprise the sugars and the starches, so by subtracting the sugar, you are left with the total starch.

For example, a can of Margaret Holmes Green & White Lima Beans contains 17g of carbohydrates and 4g of dietary fiber. If we subtract the 4g of fiber from the 17g of carbs we get 13g net carbs. The label shows there is 4g of sugars in the can of lima beans, so if we take that 4g from the 13g of net carbs we have 9g, which is the total starch per serving. We look on the label and see that a serving size is ½ cup, so you would adjust this according to how much you are planning to consume. For instance if you are planning to eat a cup of these lima beans, then you can assume there is going to be approximately 18g of starch.

The thing to remember, however, is that not all starch is "resistant starch", so it's necessary to know what foods contain resistant starches. There are quite a few different food products that contain resistant starches, but even those known to contain resistant starches have different amounts of resistant starch depending on how they are prepared.

For instance, the starch in prepared pasta is highly digestible (non-resistant) when first prepared. When you heat starch the crystalline structures amylose and amylopectin swell. When starch swells it tends to gelatinize, which makes it much more digestible.

However, when you cool pasta the structure recrystallizes such that amylase cannot get in to break the starch down into absorbable sugars, thus making it highly resistant to digestion.

It's been recently noted that if you repeat the process of cooling and heating, the crystalline structures continue to actually get tighter making it even more resistant. I would suggest, to maximize the benefit of resistant starches in pasta, you should heat it, cool it, heat it, cool it and then heat it again. This makes the resistant starches in the pasta nearly 100% resistant.

Below, I have listed some of the foods to add to your diet in order to maximize your intake of resistant starches. If you plan your meals around these foods, you should be able to exploit the greatest benefits from resistant starches while still providing yourself and your family with a wide variety of foods.

Foods High in resistant starches:

Banana (underripe): 4.7g/one medium banana

Brown rice: 1.7 g/100 g

Canned kidney beans, cooked: 2.0 g/100 g

Canned peas, cooked: 1.9 g/100 g

Canned white beans, cooked: 4.2 g/100 g

Chickpeas: 2.6 g/100 g

Cooked plantains: 3.5 g/100 g

Cooked yams: 1.5 g/100 g

Corn tortillas: 3.0 g/100 g

Cornflake cereals: 3.2 g/100 g

Fruit-filled cereal bar: 2.3 g/100 g

Italian bread, toasted: 3.8 g/100 g

Legumes: 3.3 g/100 g

Pearl barley: 2.4 g/100 g

Potatoes, cooked and cooled: 1.3 g/one medium potato

Puffed corn cereal: 1.4 g/100 g

Puffed rice cereal: 2.3 g/100 g

Puffed wheat cereal: 6.2 g/100 g

Pumpernickel bread: 4.5 g/100 g

Rolled, uncooked oats: 4.4g/100g

Rye bread: 3.2 g/100 g

Slightly green bananas: 4.7 g/one medium banana

Sourdough bread: 2.1 g/100 g

Unrolled, uncooked oats: 11.3g/100 g

Wheat pasta: 1.4 g/100 g

This is by no means a thorough list of foods containing resistant starches, however these foods contain the highest amount of resistant starch compared to most foods. RS4 (Type 4 Resistant Starches) foods may contain a much greater quantity of resistant starches, however I would not advise consuming these types of manufactured starches. It's much better to go with the whole foods that contain natural resistant starches that are balanced by vitamins and other nutrients.

One of the foods (listed above) that really packs a good supply of resistant starches is whole grain breads. Try to avoid processed foods and breads. Simply eating a couple slices of pumpernickel bread with your meals can provide 6g of resistant starches per meal, not to mention it's delicious as well, when served butter. Contrary to much popular opinion, by the way, butter is also good for you, as it contains many beneficial vitamins and recent studies show it may even actually help you in losing weight. Just don't overdo it.

A good daily diet would consist of a bowl of cornflakes for breakfast with strawberries or other fresh fruits, along with a couple pieces of whole grain toast or bread with butter, and a under-ripe banana. Perhaps a tuna sandwich on whole grain bread or a chicken pita sandwich for lunch and some good wheat pasta with pumpernickel bread (and butter) for supper. The point being you should try to include at least one resistant starch food with every meal. Experts also suggest that ¼ of the calories from every meal should consist of resistant starch with the remainder calories coming from lean protein, fruits, vegetables and health fats.

Another thing to keep in mind, if you are dieting to lose weight, is that resistant starches are great because they help you fill fuller so you don't eat as much… however don't deprive yourself too much of your favorite foods. If your favorite food is a taboo, then only eat a little bit, in moderation. If you don't allow yourself to eat your favorite foods, you'll find it much harder to stick to your diet of resistant starch and you'll be stuck in a pattern of backsliding. Go ahead, eat a couple slices of that cheesecake, or a slice or two of pizza (which actually has some resistant starch as well, if cooled and reheated)… but just don't overdo it. The added resistant starches in your diet will make up for those "bad" foods that you feel so guilty about being drawn to.

CAN RESISTANT STARCH HELP YOU LOSE WEIGHT?

Most people, when they are trying to lose weight, don't think about adding MORE starch to their diet. However, resistant starches (as we already discussed) acts quite differently than regular starches. Since resistant starches act more like fiber than traditional starches, the starches will pass through your intestines without being broken down into sugars, which are absorbed by the intestines and may end up as fat.

The reason resistant starches have helped many people lose weight is quite simply a matter of satiety. Resistant starches, increase satiety, or the feeling of being full, without increasing calories, since they are not being absorbed. This is the same effect that fiber has on your body to help in losing weight, but unlike most fibers, resistant starch is fermented in the large intestine. This fermentation creates many beneficial fatty acids, including butyrate. Butyrate actually blocks the body's ability to burn carbs. This, in turn, keeps the liver from using carbs as fuel and instead uses body fat, both stored and recently consumed, to burn for fuel.

Carbohydrates are the main source of fuel in the body, but butyrate actually prevents some of the carbs from being used as fuel, which makes your body turn to fat for it's fuel, thus literally "burning away the fat". A recent study found that if you replace only 5% of your total carbohydrates with resistant starches, the body will increase its fat burning up to 30% after a meal. It's almost the same as if your were to exercise for 30 minutes after your meal to burn the excess calories and fat.

Many studies have also found that by consuming a healthy amount of resistant starch, the body produces more satiety-inducing hormones. According to some of these studies, the balance between food intake and energy expenditure is driven by the satiety hormone called leptin. Basically, when your fat stores are full, the body produces an increase in leptin which tell the brain that we are full. If your body contains very low levels of leptin, than it is much harder to satisfy hunger, and thus we tend to eat more, adding more calories to our diet, and usually greater amounts of fat (and by virtue weight).

Another hormone that the body produces during meals is called cholecystokinin, usually abbreviated as CCK (which is much easier to say). CCK is produced in the lining of the small intestine (the duodenum or anterior intestine) and also released by some brain neurons. This hormone helps to improve digestion by slowing down the stomach's emptying of food as well as stimulating the liver's production of bile (as well as its release). bile helps the enzymes in your gut to break down fat more easily. CCK also helps to increase the fluid and enzymes from the pancreas, allowing it to break down fats, carbs and proteins more readily.

The way CCK helps with appetite suppression is by increasing the sensation of satiety in the short term during meals (as opposed to between meals). Some research has concluded that CCK does this by affecting the areas in the brain that control appetite as well as delaying the emptying of the stomach. By consuming foods high in resistant starch, the body increases production of CCK, which tells our bodies that we've eaten enough. It's been found, through several different studies, that those people who are obese (with a BMI of greater than 30) actually have a much lower level of CCK in their system. What this means is that their bodies are not producing the signals that tell them they have had enough to eat. One way to increase the production of the CCK hormone in the body is by increasing the amount of resistant starch intake, which may help go a very long way in fighting obesity, especially in those individuals who have extremely low levels of CCK, which basically means they don't feel as if they have had enough to eat, regardless of the amount of food consumed.

RESISTANT STARCH'S ROLE IN IBS & SIBO

One of the things you may have heard about Resistant Starch is that it could increase the discomforts of Irritable Bowel Syndrome (IBS) and Small Intestinal Bacterial Overgrowth (SIBO) in the small intestine. The truth is that Resistant Starch DOES have an effect on our bacteria growth, of course, so it probably will affect Irritable bowel syndrome and other bacteria problems in the intestine.

When you start including more resistant starches in your diet, the first thing most people will notices is an increase in flatulence and bloating. These usually only last for a few days and eventually will disappear in folks with a normal level of gut flora. However, people with poor gut health will notice these symptoms to an even greater degree and may have increased IBS for a week or more, depending on the level of their gut damage. You should realize, here, that we are talking about those people who already have problems with small intestinal gut bacteria and/or damage to the gut lining.

The gastrointestinal tract, which includes the small intestine, normally contains a variety of bacteria, where the greatest concentration of the bacteria is usually in the colon and much less in the small intestine. Not only is there normally a different amount of bacteria in the small intestine than in the colon, but the types of bacteria are usually different in the small intestine as well. When you have SIBO, there is an abnormally large increase in the bacteria in the small intestine and the types of bacteria are similar to the ones found in the colon.

When you start adding resistant starches to your diet, it will increase the bacteria in your gut, which (in normal circumstances) is a good thing, as this helps to produce several enzymes that help in digestion and in a healthy gut. However, if you have SIBO, then there is already an inordinate amount of bacteria in your small intestine which may impede the bacteria from reaching your gut, where it is broken down. Therefore, increasing your intake of resistant starches (as well as most fibers) will cause greater pain and discomfort to those suffering from SIBO conditions (such as Irritable Bowel Syndrome).

The controversy is whether or not you should completely avoid resistant starches if you have IBS or SIBO. Most people would say, if adding resistant starch to your diet is going to increase your discomfort, then by all means you should avoid it. However, there is some research lately, though inconclusive, that shows that by adding resistant starch to your diet, while your discomfort may increase at first, it may actually help your IBS or SIBO related ailments. in the long run. You should, in any case, start with a lower intake of resistant starch foods if you have any sort of bowel obstruction or IBS. It's recommended to take probiotics as well, to decrease the incidence of gas and bloating and help the digestive tract to break down the foods and bacteria in your intestines.

Some experts, however, believe that for short-term treatment of SIBO, antibiotics are more effective than probiotics. The problem with antibiotics is that often symptoms tend to recur after the treatment has been discontinued, requiring prolonged treatment. Prolonged usage of antibiotics can have adverse side-effects that may be even worse than the symptoms that are being treated, which makes most doctors more apt to recommend probiotics for prolonged periods, rather than antibiotics. Often, doctors will initially treat the symptoms of SIBO with antibiotics, in the short term and then use probiotics if needed for prolonged periods.

RESISTANT STARCH FOR CONSTIPATION

If you regularly suffer from constipation, you may find this chapter of Resistant Starches a real eye-opener. There are many causes of constipation, including low fiber diets, different medication, hormonal disorders and diseases that affect the colon.

Constipation is defined as fewer than three stools per week. Severe constipation is less than one stool per week. It is often accompanied by lower abdominal discomfort, hard or small stools, rectal bleeding caused by hard stools, straining to have a bowel movement and obsession with having bowel movements. It is usually caused by slower than normal movement of stools through the colon.

As we get older, the number of bowel movements generally tend to decrease. Adults may have anywhere from 3 to 21+ bowel movements per week, which is considered normal. It must be also stated that most people are irregular and may have one bowel movement on one day and 4 or 5 the next day. However, in the medical community, constipation is defined as fewer than three bowel movements per week. With this in mind, one can go without moving their bowels for 2 to 3 days without actually being constipated (medically speaking), and this should not cause any kind of physical discomfort.

Many people consider a daily bowel movement necessary to peak health, but there is actually no scientific or medical evidence to back this claim. As a matter of fact, purposely trying to move ones bowels every day, when it's not necessary can cause health problems due to straining. So, if you're not having daily bowel movements, there should be no cause for alarm as long as you are having 3 or more bowel movements per week.

If you are experiencing less than 3 bowel movements per week, you should take a look at your diet. Most causes of constipation are rooted in the diet, especially in low-fiber diets, but medications have also been shown to be a culprit in many cases. Narcotics, antidepressants and anticonvulsants are amongst the chief medications known to cause constipation, along with iron supplements and Calcium channel blocking (CCBs) drugs such as Cardizem and Procardia. Constipation arising from the use of these drugs can usually be treated quite easily by the introduction of increased fiber and resistant starches in your diet.

It is important, however, to distinguish between acute constipation and chronic constipation. Acute (or sudden onset) constipation should be checked immediately as there may be an underlying medical illness that is causing the constipation, such as tumors of the colon. If you experience rectal bleeding, severe abdominal pains or cramps, nausea or vomiting, you should also consider seeing a healthcare professional as soon as possible to rule out any serious underlying condition.

However, chronic (or long term) constipation may not be as urgent, as long as the aforementioned symptoms are not accompanying the constipation, especially when a simple change in diet can provide relief.

By consuming foods that are known to be high in Resistant Starches, the carbohydrates in the food resists digestion in the small intestines and is moved along to the colon (or large intestine) where it begins to break down (or ferment). This fermentation process helps to stimulate production of the good bacterias in our guts.

As mentioned earlier, the bacteria produced by this fermentation process are called propionic, acetic and butyric acids. It is these three SCFA's (Short-Chain-Fatty-Acids) that help to improve the gastrointestinal barrier function. Butyric Acid has even been shown to improve the motility of the gut, which helps to decrease abdominal pain during defecation. Normally, butyric acid is quickly absorbed by the small intestine, but with Resistant Starches, this acid is quickly moved along to the colon, with little absorption, which allow the colon to make use of it in a much greater capacity. Some studies have shown that butyric acids help to increase gut contractions, which helps to move stools and increase the bulk of those stools.

The bacteria produced by the aforementioned SCFAs also play an important part in increasing pH in the colon, allowing it to be more acidic. This, in turn, helps to improve your gut health and helps to decrease the risk of leaky gut as well as helping to increase your body's ability to break down foods, thus increasing the movement of stools.

One thing that's important to keep in mind, when you are adding resistant starch to your diet, especially when you are suffering from constipation, is to add the right kind of resistant starch. We covered the 4 different types of resistant starches back in chapter 4, but I want to briefly touch on the types again here, as it relates to gut health and constipation.

RS1 - Found in grains seeds and legumes, may cause more digestions problems in many people and probably isn't a good choice if you are suffering constipation or have other digestive ailments.

RS2 - Found in green bananas, raw plantains and raw white potatoes are not very digestible (or edible for that matter) and should be avoided if you are suffering from any kind of digestive problems, though unrefined potato starch powder is an excellent source of resistant starch for digestive issues.

RS3 - Retrograde resistant starch is the starch that forms after RS2 or RS1 starches have been allowed to cool. This means if you cook and cool potatoes, rice, legume, etc. You get RS3 which is excellent type for those suffering with constipation and other types of digestive disorders.

RS4 - Industrial Resistant Starch is chemically modified, man-made starch, usually made in the powder form. This starch never occurs naturally and for this reason alone, it is probably a good idea to avoid it. It has been shown to be mostly ineffective against constipation and other related gut problems. Hi-Maize is an example of this type of Resistant Starch.

As you can see, the best Resistant Starch for constipation (and most other stomach ailments) would be RS3. RS2 in the form of potato powder is great, but be sure that you get the unrefined potato starch powder with no added chemicals or modifications. Retrograde Starch (or RS3) is the easiest to get and the best source I have found for fighting digestion problems.

Getting RS3 starch is simply a matter of cooking, cooling and reheating starchy carbs. You should cook your carbs as you normally would, this includes rice, potatoes, polenta, lentils, peas and split peas, pasta, carrots, sweet potatoes, etc. Allow the food to cool to room temperature (if you are going to eat it soon) or put it in the refrigerator for later use. You can serve it cold, and still get a good supply of RS3, but if you reheat it, you get even more RS3. If you want the maximum amount of resistant starch from these foods, try cooking them, cooling them, reheating them, cooling them and reheating them again.

By cooling these starches you are converting the carbs (which is made mostly of digestible starch) into resistant starch (indigestible starch). It's called resistant starch because of how the starch resists the normal enzymes in your gut that breaks carbs down and release glucose into your bloodstream, which causes blood sugar to surge.

Researches have found that by eating cold pasta, many people experience much smaller spikes in their glucose levels as opposed to eating cooked pasta. The results were even more dramatic in those who cooled and then reheated the pasta. As a matter of fact the cooled and cooked pasta was shown to reduce glucose spikes by as much as 50%. This means, not only will you be helping to reduce the onset or duration of constipation, but you will be helping to reduce blood glucose spikes which can cause many unwanted health issues, including diabetes.

Many studies have shown that freshly cooked legumes, grains and tubers (such as potatoes) contained a significantly higher amount of Resistant Starches when cooked, cooled and recooked several times. As a matter of fact, the Resistant Starch in peas were shown to increase over 110%!! So if you want to get the most out of your foods, in the form of resistant starch, you should cook, cool, cook cool, cook cool (you get the idea). You should repeat the process at least 2 or 3 times for maximum RS.

RESISTANT STARCH & LEAKY GUT SYNDROME

Leaky Gut Syndrome (or Intestinal Permeability) is a common condition affecting literal tens of thousands of people a year. Many of our modern autoimmune disorders can be linked to this problem, including IBS, Crohn's Disease, Multiple Sclerosis, Addison's Disease, Chronic Fatigue Syndrome, Lupus, Fibromyalgia and Asthma. It's also been found to be a chief cause of things such as allergies and food sensitivities, chemical sensitivities and even thyroiditis.

Leaky Gut Syndrome is hardly talked about in the media, yet it's a condition that can cause many health problems. There are many people who have a Leaky Gut and are totally unaware of it. "Leaky Gut" refers to a gut that has become inflamed and very porous. This allows large food proteins as well as fungi, bacteria and toxic substances to be absorbed right into the bloodstream.

Ordinarily the walls of the intestinal are considered semi permeable, which means that pores allow only specific things to enter the bloodstream while blocking other things from entering the bloodstream. Vitamins and minerals are absorbed from the foods you eat by small microscopic pores found in the small intestine. These nutrients are then transferred into the bloodstream where they are carried to the different organs by the blood. However, toxins and large undigested food particles are blocked from being absorbed into the bloodstream, normally.

When the gut becomes "leaky" it causes these intestinal pores to widen, which then allows undigested food particles and toxins to enter into the bloodstream instead of being blocked. When such foreign objects enter into the bloodstream, it causes the immune system to attack them, which often leads to allergies.

Basically what is happening is that your immune system sees these foreign particles and recognizes a danger, thus setting up an immune response and building up antibodies to protect us from them. The big problem here is that the body doesn't only build up these antibodies to the food particles, but it also attacks the healthy cells. This leads to inflammation and cause many symptoms such as:

- Bloating
- Fatigue
- Headaches
- Joint Pain
- Food Sensitivities
- Digestive Problems
- Weight Gain
- and many other symptoms

One of the most notable signs of leaky gut is food sensitivity. When your body realizes there are foreign particles seeping into it, as stated above, it goes on the attack and will set up a defense against those food particles, thus causing "food allergies". This doesn't mean you'll break out in hives, or that you will swell up, but it can lead to any of the symptoms listed above, as well as Arthritis, psoriasis, chronic fatigue syndrome, migraines, muscle pains, depression and anxiety (to name a few). There is also some strong evidence that leaky gut can even lead to Type 1 Diabetes, according to the Journal of Diabetes.

While there is much evidence that Resistant Starch will stave off leaky gut syndrome, unfortunately Resistant Starch cannot cure leaky gut. If you already are suffering from leaky gut then you will want to get it under control before beginning an intake of resistant starches, as resistant starches can actually exacerbate the issue. However, there are many different ways you can help heal leaky gut, including a daily intake of bone broth, coconut oil and other coconut products, fermented vegetables such as sauerkraut and kimchi, eating more steamed vegetables and foods rich in Omega-3 all help to heal the leaky gut.

One of the most important things you should do in order to heal your leaky gut is to cut out those foods that might damage and inflame your gut lining. It may take several months for your gut to fully heal, but until it is fully healed, you would do very well to stay away from grains, legumes and most dairy products, (though some people may tolerate ghee). You should also try to avoid any kind of food additives such as found in most processed foods, and try to stick with whole foods. Some vegetable may also cause irritation such as eggplants, tomatoes, potatoes and peppers.

Not only is it important to cut out those foods that may further irritate your gut, but also try to eat more foods that can reduce the inflammation as well. Try to decrease foods rich in omega-6 and increase your intake of foods rich in Omega-3. Omega-6 foods include vegetable oils, meat from grain-fed animals and most nuts and seeds. All of these foods tend to increase inflammation, whereas foods that contain Omega-3, such as meat from pasture fed animals, free-range eggs, and wild fish are great for reducing inflammation.

You should also eat a variety of vegetables, going for a full range of colors, to help control inflammation. Make sure to steam the vegetables well so they are broken down more easily by your digestive system. You should also try to eat the dark green vegetables daily as well to provide the essential vitamins and minerals your body needs in a way that's easier to absorb.

If you have leaky gut, the chances are you need more healthy gut microflora, in which case probiotics should be an essential part of your diet. You can add probiotics to your diet, either in supplemental form or through foods. This will increase the good bacteria and get rid of the bad, in order to facilitate the healing of the gut lining. Some natural ways to get a good dose of probiotics is through foods such as unpasteurized sauerkraut and other unpasteurized fermented vegetables. Kombucha tea is also an excellent source of probiotics as is coconut milk yoghurt or kefir.

As your gut begins to heal, you should try to provide the body with plenty of proteins, vitamins and minerals as well as "good" fats. Wild caught fish and meat from grass-fed animals and plenty of healthy vegetables are an essential way to help to heal that leaky gut, and don't forget the coconut and bone broth.

Medium chain saturated fats are also very gentle on the lining of your gut and be absorbed easily, without having to be broken down by digestive enzymes, therefore providing you with a good source of energy without any type of modification. This is very helpful in healing the lining of your gut. Bone Broth is one excellent source, regardless of what source of animal used. Chicken, duck, lamb, pork and fish are all anti-microbial, anti-inflammatory and have many key nutrients to help rebuild your gut lining. Bone broth is also rich in the amino acids proline and glycine, which helps regulate digestion and reduce inflammation, as well as healing almost every part of the body.

Taking digestive enzyme supplements at the beginning of your meals will also help in fully digesting the food so that less particles are leaked out of the gut.

Once you have gotten your leaky gut under control, then it's a great time to start adding resistant starch to your diet, in order to maximize the health of your gut and minimize the recurrence of the leaky gut. Start out with small doses of resistant starch, particularly the RS3 type, until your body gets used to it. Some bloating and discomfort may occur at first, but these symptoms should disappear with a few days. Above all else, if you suspect you are suffering from leaky gut see your healthcare provider immediately (preferably an holistic healthcare provider) to be sure there are not other conditions that have been or are being produced by the leaky gut.

RESISTANT STARCH FOR DIABETES

It has been estimated that over 25 million children and adults in the US have diabetes, which equates to a health cost of about $218 Billion. The most common strategies for fighting diabetes is lifestyle intervention, mainly modulations to your dietary intake.

Dietary fibers have been used, traditionally, for managing blood glucose levels and, according to the National Institute of Health dietary fiber has been linked to improved glycemic control in those with diabetes as well as healthy individuals.

Resistant starch has been shown to have a significant effect on insulin sensitivity as well as fatty acid metabolism, however, the efficacy of Resistant Starch in individuals with Type 2 Diabetes has not been thoroughly investigated. Animal studies, however, have shown that Resistant Starch improves glucose and insulin metabolism through increased postprandial secretion by stimulating the colonic enteroendocrine cells within the intestines.

While the research is still fairly new, more scientists and medical specialists are discovering a link between resistant starch and diabetes. While resistant starches are carbohydrates, unlike starch and sugar resistant starch and fiber will help to stabilize glucose rather than raise it.

The quicker your body digests carbohydrates, the faster it produces glucose. The faster your body produces glucose, the higher your blood sugar will rise. This is why basic sugars and starches have such a dramatic impact on your blood sugar level, as they are easily digested. By eating foods that are not so easily digested, you can help stabilize your glucose levels. Resistant starch is one food that is very slowly digested, thus helping you to keep your blood sugars steady.

An added benefit of eating resistant starch to help stabilize glucose levels is that it helps by making you feel fuller quicker (satiety), which helps to stave off hunger for a longer time, leading to less calorie consumption. Which means there are less in-between meal snacks, which helps further in keeping your glucose level.

While it's true that resistant starch slows your digestion and helps to stabilize your glucose level, if you have diabetes you must consider your overall carbohydrate intake as well. Bananas, Potatoes and corn starches will raise your glucose levels, so you should avoid these foods, even though they are high in resistant starch. You want to choose foods that are lower on the glycemic index such as barley, lentils and other legume and oatmeal.

The glycemic index measures the potential of certain foods to raise your glucose levels. Foods that are less than 55 on the glycemic level have a minimum impact on your body's sugar levels.

Most diabetics are warned to carefully count their carbs, and many have been taught that ALL carbohydrates (with the exception of fiber) are to be avoided as they easily break down into sugar in the small intestine. However, resistant starch is a carbohydrate that isn't easily digested, and only recently has the medical community started waking up to the fact that resistant starches can be added to the diabetic diet. Not only does resistant starch resist digestion, but as it leaves the small intestine (pretty much intact) and moves onto the large intestine, the resistant starch is fermented by the bacteria and short-chain fatty acids are then formed.

These short-chain fatty acids play a big role in our overall health including:

- Promoting colon health
- Lowering blood glucose levels
- Lowering blood cholesterol levels
- Reducing appetite
- Boosting the immune system

One study has shown that people who replace a certain percentage of their carbohydrates with Resistant Starch had between 20% and 30% higher fat oxidation after a meal. This means that subjects on Resistant Starch burned fat faster than those who simply took in other carbohydrates. As mentioned previously throughout this book, the short-chain fatty acid, butyrate appears to block the body's ability to turn carbohydrates into fuel so that the body instead tends to burn more fat.

There is actually no Recommended Daily Allowance for Resistant Starch (at least not yet) but many experts have estimated that our typical resistant starch intake should be at least 4 grams per day. I would suggest at least 3 times or more of that amount, as it's not hard to do and you will see the benefits more rapidly.

Studies have indicated that between 15 and 30 grams of resistant starch (equivalent to about 2 to 4 tablespoons of potato starch) was the most beneficial. In one study, different amounts of resistant starch was given to several subjects. The results were that those who consumed the most resistant starches showed improved insulin sensitivity (especially in the overweight and obese) with approximately 10% of body weight reduction.

In chapter 5 we listed some foods with their resistant starch content. I would suggest you look over that chart and find the foods you enjoy the most, as well as those containing the highest concentration of Resistant Starch and then begin incorporating those foods into your daily diet regimen.

If you are diabetic and have chosen to supplement your diet with Resistant starch, it is highly recommended that you start with small amounts t begin with and gradually increase that amount as your body builds up a tolerance to resistant starch. Remember, as stated in previous chapters, you may feel some bloating and experience an increase in gas at first, and this is to be expected due to the way the bacteria is being broken down and your gut flora is changing. If you feel a marked discomfort after a few days, then you should decrease the amount, then gradually increase until you are feeling no discomfort or very little discomfort.

If you are experiencing quite a bit of discomfort even with small amounts of Resistant Starch, then this may be an indication of SIBO, which we have briefly covered in chapter 7. It could also be an indication of microbial dysbiosis (or an imbalance of microbial bacteria). It is recommended that you consult with a healthcare practitioner if you find that even the smallest amount of resistant starches to have a negative impact on you. A good holistic healthcare professional can help you balance gut microbiome through antimicrobials and probiotics. Once you have this balance, then you should be able to easily take resistant starch with little or no discomfort.

CONCLUSION

In this book we have taken the mystery out of carbohydrates, what they are and how they work. Now you can actually talk about carbs and know what you are talking about. We also touched on fiber and where it comes from and how it's utilized. Of course fiber is a very important part of your diet and easily obtained from most roughage, as well as breads and cereals. We then learned about the differences between fiber and starch. Many people don't even realize there is a difference, whereas others believe fiber is good and starch is bad. By now you should realize that starch can be a good thing or bad, depending on how you get your starch.

You have learned, finally, what resistant starches are and how they work almost the same way as fiber to keep your digestive track healthy and your gut bacterial happy and working properly. You've discovered that resistant starch, also called a third fiber and often regarded as "dietary fiber" works to keep you healthy and free from many diseases, but also helps to make you feel full, which in turn helps you to eat less and lose weight.

We've also touched upon IBS, SIBO, Leaky Gut and Diabetes and the effects resistant starch might have on these conditions as well. I would like to point out that by increasing your intake of resistant starch now, you can avoid these and other serious health problems in the future. If you already have one or more of these conditions, it would be a good idea to see your healthcare professional before attempting to drastically change your diet or take on more resistant starches. Your healthcare professional may advise you to hold off on the resistant starch until your microbiome flora in your gut has been balanced through the use of probiotics or antibiotics (depending on your condition)

We covered quite a bit of territory in a very small space, and it will probably behoove you to go over this short book several times, to let everything sink in, but once you have gotten the basics you are well on your way of becoming a resistant starch guru, able to plan your meals around resistant starches to maximize your health and well-being. This book has gone beyond simply telling you what foods are good for you and what foods to avoid, but has given you the ability to understand why the foods containing resistant starch are as good as many dieticians and nutritional experts say they are.

Like the old adage goes give a man a fish, he will eat for a day. Teach a man to fish, he will eat for a lifetime. You have been given the tools to understand how to "fish" out the best foods for their nutritional value, you have been shown where to go and what to look for, even to reading labels in order to allow you to break down how much starch is in those resistant starch foods, through simple mathematics. Some day (hopefully) the USDA will begin adding resistant starches to our food labels to make it easier for you to pick out the best foods for yourself and your family, but until that day comes, you can still do it yourself by following the method outlines in the last chapter.

Finally, I would like to restate that if you are trying to lose weight (as well as keeping yourself healthier) you cannot go wrong with a resistant starch diet, try to eat at least one food per meal that contains resistant starch. Don't forget, to allow yourself treats as well, so that you don't feel deprived and end up going off your good diet and back to unhealthy eating. If you give yourself a treat once in a while, you'll find it much easier to stick with your resistant starch regime. Just make sure on your next shopping trip, to stock up on those foods we've outlined and when you are cooking that delicious pasta, do be sure to cool it at least twice before eating it to maximize those resistant starches. A resistant starch diet should not be limiting or a chore, as you have a plethora of foods to choose from...just be sure to choose the right foods, then mix them up and eat them down.

Bon Appétit!

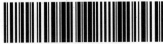

19544384R00029

Printed in Great Britain
by Amazon